ISBN-13:
978-1503307377

ISBN-10:
1503307379

Library of Congress Control Number:
2014921016
CreateSpace Independent Publishing
Platform, North Charleston, SC

DEATH, BURIAL, RESURRECTION

BY: DAMIEN ISHAMEL FAIRCONETUE

Chapter 1

IF MY PEOPLE

Ali and Allie are riding the city bus to the library. Allie is sitting in the seat closest to the window. Ali is sitting next to her. They pass other people walking on the sidewalks, driving vehicles and going in and out of stores. The time is 12:00pm. It is lunchtime for most people. Allie is a nurse at Grace and Mercy Hospital. She works the graveyard shift from 11:00pm to 7:00am. She is going to the library with Ali. Ali is a college student. He is a history major but has no definite career plans. They are friends, but Ali wants more from his relationship with Allie. Ali and Allie are in New Orleans. The city is fast-moving, and the people are fast talkers. Ali and Allie find it hard to maintain the pace sometimes. Nonetheless, they're fast enough to survive. The bus stops at the library, and a few, other people with Ali and Allie walk off the bus. Ali lets Allie walk ahead of him. Ali and Allie walk side by side as equals into the library. Ali loves to do research on various subjects of history. He is researching the history of diseases and the man-made remedies for it.

The library has two floors, so Ali and
Allie use an elevator to go to the
second floor. Allie finds a book about
religion and sits on the sofa to read
it. On the other hand, Ali walks up
and down a few aisles until he comes
across a hardcover book with thick
pages. Ali gets the book from the
shelf and walks back to Allie. Ali
sits beside her, opens the book and
begins to read it.

Ali said, "Reading books is like
reading people. We have a lot of
knowledge in us if we can just get past
the hardcover."

Allie replied, "I like books with
soft covers. Soft covers are less
intimidating. I like books with soft
covers and colorful faces."

Ali said, "However, hard covers
are needed for books with thick pages.
Hard covers can support the weight of
heavier books."

Allie replied, "That is true.
Just like a strong man can support a
woman with a lot of burdens."

Ali asked, "Burdens? Like what?"

Allie replied, "A wife is as the
weaker vessel. Everybody needs
somebody to lean on."

Ali said, "Like the song, 'Lean on
Me'."

Ali and Allie began to sing "Lean
on Me" just loud enough, so they could
hear one another.

By the way, this is a library, and people are supposed to be quiet. Other people are here to do some serious studying.

Allie said, "That sounded good. We make good music together."

Ali asked, "Yeah, we do. Allie, have you ever considered us as a couple instead of just friends?

Allie replied, "One time. I like you as a friend, but I will enjoy you as a lover."

Ali asked, "Can friends enjoy one another?"

Allie replied, "Sure. Lovers are friends first. When the joy is gone, the love stops."

Ali said, "That's true. My parents were lovers. But, their marriage became a grievous burden instead of a joyous relationship. They began to do things for one another out of obligation instead of for the pure intent to see the other one happy."

Allie replied, "Yeah. How does this make you feel as their son?"

Ali answered, "I feel torn. I love my parents. I refuse to take sides in their arguments. I just leave them alone and come to a place like this or go to you."

Allie asked, "So, you find comfort in me?"

Ali replied, "Yeah. You're less intimidating, and your appearance is more colorful."

Allie asked, "Ali, are you comparing me to a book?"

Ali replied, "We are all books."

Allie said, "I might look soft and pretty, but I have a lot of issues that you would not think I have."

Ali asked, "Like what?"

Allie replied, "Not here. This is a public place. We have to be alone with God for me to open myself to you in this way. I'm not talking about sexually but psychologically. Before a man can take on my body, he must take on my mind. I mean that before a man can make love to me, he has to understand me."

Ali said, "I feel you on that, sister. You have a right to feel and be secure in any relationship. Do you feel some security with me?"

Allie replied, "Yes. Ali, you and I have known each other for a while, and trust has been built between us to make our relationship strong."

Ali asked, "So, are you ready to take this thing to the next level?"

Allie replied, "You mean, being intimate?

Ali said, "Yeah. One day."

Allie replied, "Let me allow you to know what's in my mind. What makes me happy, sad and mad. Are you willing to walk this distance?"

Ali said, "Sure. I know it won't be easy. Nothing worth having is easy to get but it is worth it. And, you are worth all the hell that I have to endure to receive you."

Allie replied, "I'm not going to put you through hell. I'm not the devil or some, other women that provoke men to anger and leave them so distressed enough to kill other people."

Ali said, "I know you are not a devil or any of these, other women. I know that you value our friendship as much as I value it, and you will never do anything to hurt me."

Allie replied, "I'm glad that you know this, Ali, because I love you."

Ali put his right arm around Ali and moved close to her face to kiss her. Allie turned her face to Ali to kiss him. They kissed for a few minutes.

Ali said, "That felt good. I dreamed of kissing you for a long time."

Allie replied, "Really. It feels good to be wanted especially by a friend like you, Ali."

Ali said, "I love you, Allie."

Allie replied, "I love you, too."

Chapter 2

WHICH ARE CALLED BY MY NAME

The church has been a sanctuary
for troubled people in an evil world.
In saying this, the church is full of
compassion. God calls them pitiful.
Pitiful does not mean miserable but
full of pity. At Salvation Holiness
Church, the people help one another.
Nobody is rich, but everybody has what
he or she needs. Ali invited Allie to
a church service one Sunday morning.
This is not a big church. It is the
size of a shotgun house in a low to
medium-income neighborhood. However,
the building is full of people. The
windows are clear with no stained
glass. Pastor Clark does not want
God's people to have a delusional image
about the world from the church. He
wants them to see the world as it is.
In addition, Pastor Clark teaches
people to see themselves as they are
and make the necessary changes for the
better. Nonetheless, Ali and Allie are
sitting on a pew ¾ the way to the back
of the sanctuary. The people are
lively. The choir sings Amazing Grace,
Swing Low; Sweet Chariot and other
Negro spirituals. Nonetheless, a few
Caucasian people attend the worship
services also. Allie is sitting inside
Ali.

Ali's right arm rests on the back of the pew around Allie in order to let the world know that "this one's mine." The congregation shows their approval to the choir by the tapping of their shoes, standing and singing with the choir, waving their hands, shouting hallelujahs and amen's, dancing, speaking in tongues and kneeling at the altar. This happens for several minutes until everyone praises the grief out of them. Then, the choir stops singing, musicians stop playing and people sit in order to prepare to receive the bread of life from the man of God. Furthermore, Pastor Clark stands behind the pulpit and opens the Holy Bible on the podium. Pastor Clark stands about 6'2" and is medium built. He is a man of dark complexion and a deep voice. Nonetheless, Pastor's Clark's spirit is smooth and gentle like blessed oil.

Pastor Clark said, "Good morning, church, and praise the Lord."

Church said, "Praise the Lord."

Pastor Clark said, "Let us pray. Our Father in Heaven, thank you. Thank you for life, health and well being. Speak to us, and prepare our hearts to receive your word, Lord. Amen."

Church said, "Amen."

Pastor Clark said, "Can you please stand for the reading of the Word of God?"

The church stands with their
Bibles open in their hands.

Pastor Clark said, "The message
comes from St.Luke 5:32. And, it
reads. Jesus says, 'I came not to call
the righteous but sinners to
repentance. You may be seated. Thank
you."

The church sits in their seats.
The attention is focused on the man of
God.

Pastor Clark said, "What is a
revival? A revival is not a social
gathering, fund-raising event or pep
rally. A revival is the working of
miracles and special miracles. The
working of miracles is one of the gifts
of the Holy Spirit. Special miracles
come from God also. Special miracles
are the resurrection of the dead. We
cannot conjure revivals. Revivals
happen when the people believe in Jesus
Christ. Jesus Christ is the Word of
God. In the beginning was the Word.
And, the Word was with God, and the
Word was God. Jesus the Son is the
Word made flesh. God is a Spirit. To
clarify, JEHOVAH, the Spirit of God, is
the gift. Jesus the Man is the gift
box and wrapping. When you receive
Jesus, you receive JEHOVAH. When you
receive JEHOVAH, you receive Jesus.
You cannot get to JEHOVAH without Jesus
because JEHOVAH is in Jesus.

To illustrate, our spirits are in us; but we are known by the name of our flesh. God is known to us by Jesus. He is the perfect image of God. Let's get back to revival.

One other man shouted, "That's alright, pastor. Preach."

Pastor Clark replied, "2 Chronicles 7:14 states, 'If my people which are called by my name-'. God's name is Jesus Christ. He calls us to repentance. Therefore, God is talking to us. 'Shall humble themselves and pray'-. Just like we put our lives in the human doctors' hands in order to do surgeries in us, we must put our lives in God's hands in order to do surgeries in us. 'and pray-'. Prayer is death or the surrendering of our powers to God. Humility is the agreement to put our lives in God's hands. Prayer is the actual surrender. 'And seek my face-'. Calling on the name of the Lord in our weakness and surrender to his divine will is seeking His face. God is a Spirit. He cannot be seen in the natural. We must die in order to see God's face. 'And turn from their wicked ways-'. Every idea that comes from people but does not heal us is wicked. Therefore, drugs are wicked. We must go to the best doctor in order to get the best care.

'Then will I hear from heaven-'. The answer to HIV/AIDS, Ebola and Cancer is in Jesus. May the Lord bless you with these words."

The church stands, claps their hands and shouts, 'Hallelujah'. Then, the choir stands and begins to sing, 'This is the day that the Lord has made.' Everybody is full of joy. Some people are crying and laughing while they are singing. Deacon Watson stands before the congregation and begins to speak with a microphone in his right hand.

Deacon Watson said, "They that wait on the Lord shall renew their strength. I tell you, church. Wait on Him. God's time is greater than our times. Our times are 12-hour and 24-hour clocks and a 12-month calendar. God does not work according to our times. He is going to heal our loved ones. He will heal us. I say if we believe, we shall see the glory of God. I have been a doctor for 20 years and have never seen a power like God's. Wait on Him. Wait on Him. Wait on Him."

The Church declared, "Yes."

Several, other people started to dance, shout and speak in tongues. This is a glorious time, but the glory has not come yet. This is in anticipation of the glory.

Chapter 3
SHALL HUMBLE THEMSELVES AND PRAY

Allie struggled with a sickness that she concealed from everybody else for a while. To the contrary, Allie believed God. In addition, Allie believed in God. Allie knew that the human doctors could not cure the condition or heal her. Nonetheless, Allie remembered the scripture that her grandfather reminded her many times during his troubles. The verse is 2 Chronicles 7:14. Allie lies on her bed with her face to Heaven. Allie's strength continues to leave her body a little at a time daily. Allie frowns and becomes frustrated with God's plan to cure this condition and heal her. Suddenly, Ali knocks on her door.

Ali said, "Allie, good morning. It's me, Ali."

Allie replied, "Come on in, baby. I'm in the bed."

Ali opens the door, walks into Allie's apartment and upstairs into her bedroom. Ali sits on the bed next to Allie.

Ali asked, "Are you better?"

Allie replied, "No. I prayed to God to make me better. But, I don't know what's happening."

Ali said, "Remember the woman with the issue of blood from the Bible."

"The doctors could not cure the condition or heal her. Nonetheless, she trusted in the Lord Jesus Christ. She agreed to touch the hem of Jesus' garment in order to be made whole. The Bible is God's word. God's time is greater than ours because He is greater than we are. Our times are 12 or 24-hour clocks and a 12-month calendar. God does not work according to our times. He is the doctor with the most knowledge, skills and experience. Nonetheless, that woman had a blood condition. The blood is the life of the flesh, and life is in the blood. Therefore, the blood can infect the rest of the body if it is infected. Hence, in order to cure an aggressive sickness, Jesus lets the sickness run its course in order to exhaust its strength. Then, it will not have anymore strength to fight; it will surrender. In addition, the Lord stops the creation of blood cells and waits for the remaining ones to dry up in the body. This is what you are feeling. The Lord is not only a doctor. He is also a surgeon. He shall put you to sleep, open your flesh and let your body dry out in order to purge the cause of the sickness and cure the condition.

Next, the Lord will put new cells into your body, heal your body and circulate the cells to run blood through your body for its regeneration. After you are regenerated, Jesus will resurrect you."

Allie replied slowly, "I am the resurrection and the life. He that believes in me; though he were dead, yet shall he live. Ali, I see a huge snake ascending before me. Who is He?"

Ali said, "Moses lifted a model serpent of metal before the sick people to behold for their health. This serpent is Jesus Christ, Allie. Look to Him. Jesus works like a hypothermic needle. He takes out the bad blood, let you sleep for a little while and put good blood into you."

Allie replied, "Yes, Ali. I am naturally afraid of snakes, but this one is different. He is meek and gentle. His fangs hurt just for a little bit, and I do feel the blood slowly coming out of my body. Because, I am weak and want to sleep. But, I love you, Ali. I want a life with you."

Ali said, "And you will have a life with me. I love you, too. I'll be here in this waiting room called Earth until the Lord brings you out of surgery."

Allie replied, "Thank you, baby. Thank you, Jesus."

13

Ali continues to hold Allie's right hand in both of his hands. Ali leans over to Allie's face and kisses her on the lips.

Ali said, "No sickness or disease is going to keep me from loving you, Allie."

Ali sits back upright and keeps his eyes on Allie. Allie keeps her eyes on Ali. Then, Allie drifts into a deep sleep that we know as death. Ali begins to cry and feel sorrow for the temporary loss of his friend's company. Nevertheless, Ali remembers what Jesus tells Martha.

Jesus says in Ali's mind, "I am the resurrection and the life. He that believes in me, though he were dead; yet shall he live. If you would believe, Ali, you should see the glory of God."

However, it is difficult for Ali to put a smile on his face, but he thinks back to what he tells Allie about God's time and human time. In saying this, the Bible is written in a time-condensed form, so we can understand it. Nevertheless, the Bible is God's word. Therefore, it is originally in God's time. Ali continues to attend classes in order to pursue his degree, but he has another mission in life.

Hence, Ali prepares speeches and pamphlets to explain the healing power of Jesus Christ to everybody else that he meets. This is what motivates him to keep going. Without Jesus, Ali would follow Allie into the grave. Ali has faith. Ali is fighting the good fight of faith. In addition, it is a tumultuous battle in his mind. Ali has peace only in his sleep, and it is too short in his opinion. However, Ali can't stop moving. Ali grieves for Allie, but he hopes for the manifestation of the promise of Jesus Christ. Every now and then, God sends angels to Ali that give him messages of hope in special miracles and a better life with Allie. One day, Ali opens his Bible to St. John 11. He reads that Jesus raises Lazarus from the dead, and many; other people believe on God for this. However, the religious, non-Christian community criticizes the works of God and makes plans to kill Jesus. Then, Jesus decides to walk no more openly with the people but to dwell in Ephraim with His disciples. Ali begins to preach to himself and rejoice in his spirit. However, Ali shows concern outwardly in anticipation of the many attacks that might come from Satan in order to make Ali's life as miserable as Satan can make it. Nonetheless, Ali continues to live.

Chapter 4
AND SEEK MY FACE

Ali is sitting on the floor in his apartment. The lights are off, and it is evening. Ali is sitting against the wall and bearing all his weight on it. Ali is fighting the good fight of faith. He is frustrated with the loss of his friend, Allie. Nonetheless, Ali is reminded about the promises of God.

Ali said, "I know that you don't get joy from your people's suffering but from their salvation. The book of Job is not about people's suffering but about you looking for a Savior for your people. Lord, I know that you are in me; but, I want to see you around me. I want to see you in other people. The world has many friends. Many people comfort them. However, I am alone. If it is not too much to ask, can you give me Christian friends? I don't want these fake tail people from the man-made churches. They put on just a show in order to get my money. They have no compassion. They don't believe in miracles much less special miracles. However, they believe in financial miracles. It's all about money to them.

Most of the preachers are part of
multi-billion dollar faith-based
enterprises, so they don't have to work
a daily job like other people work. No
wonder they can say, 'praise God.' I
give them all this money, and they
won't visit me in the hospital.
They'll send somebody else. However,
some of them preach the truth; but they
don't have the compassion of the truth.
Don't they know that compassion comes
before miracles? Even you, LORD, pity
your people. You have compassion on
us. You feel for our misfortunes, but
these pulpit pimps feel for nothing but
the money in our pockets. I love you,
Lord Jesus. I believe in you, the
Father, Son and Holy Spirit. I believe
in the gifts of the Spirit, but I don't
have the time for games anymore. I
'don had enough. It's people that live
like the devil in hell, and they have
more material possessions than I have.
But, they don't have the faith that I
have. They don't hear from God like I
hear from you. They won't be prepared
to see the special miracles or go back
with you into Heaven. I just feel
miserable as a Christian. Being a
Christian in this world is a miserable
existence.

Nonetheless, your word says that 'great gain is contentment.' It's just hard to be content but see other people with the things that I desire. Is it wrong to have a successful business? Is it wrong to own a house? Lord, you can trust me with nice things. I won't get the big head. I won't become arrogant. I won't forget my past. These false prophets are on the payrolls in multi-billion dollar faith-based enterprises. They don't have to fight with the devil like I have to fight. They get everything they want without struggles, or it seems this way. Looks can be deceiving, however. I am lonely, Jesus. I know that you are with me, but I am still lonely in the flesh. Make me a help mate for me. I'll wait on my wife. I'll wait on Allie to return to me. Other people think that it is the grief and depression talking through me, but I know your word. Am I the only person that believes your word, Lord Jesus? I don't want to be the only one that believes your word. If this is true, it is a lonely world. I find peace only during sleep. I wish that I can sleep forever. I'm sorry, Lord. Wishing is for sinners, but praying is for saints. Nevertheless, I'm not suicidal. I won't hurt myself or other people, but I am lonely.

Nobody else wants to listen to me
because they say, 'you're having a pity
party.' They don't even know what pity
means. You tell us, Lord Jesus, to be
pitiful or full of compassion because
you are pitiful. I'm talking to you
like you are real, God, because you are
real. Answer me like a real God
answers. I'm tired of having
misfortunes follow me like a chain
connected to a collar around my neck.
If I try to work to succeed or have
success, something always happens to
take this success away and bring me
back down. I love you, Lord Jesus, but
sometimes, I hate being a Christian in
this world. I guess loving you and
being a Christian is not based on
feeling, but love is a spirit. Love is
a power, a constant power that exists
with all feelings. It's like Allie and
I. We loved one another even when we
were mad and happy at one another.
Here I am, a child of the great King.
And, I'm running from boisterous women
that attack me for Allie's sickness.
How does this look, Lord? I'm just
like Elijah. Well, I know one thing.
Elijah went up to Heaven, but Jezebel
died a violent death in the end. This
is the world I live. I live in a God-
hating, Christ-hating, man-hating
world.

So, where do I begin to look for you, Jesus? You are a Spirit. You cannot be found in things. Therefore, in order to find you, I must leave myself. I must leave my body. I must leave the light of this life and go into the darkness of the next life. You are the light on the candlestick in the dark room of paradise. You spoke to Moses in dark speeches. You spoke to Moses from the spirit world. I cannot be afraid to leave my comfort zone in order to seek your face. In this darkness, I will find faith. I will be able to see what you are doing and will manifest before it comes to the natural. Little children are afraid of the dark, but I must man-up and look into this darkness in order to see your light from afar. If I come near to you, you will come near to me. I will be like Moses, the meekest man in the earth. Gang members claim they have knowledge, but they have knowledge according to this world. They will perish with the knowledge of this world because everything in this world will be destroyed by fire. Nonetheless, I'll wait on you, Lord. I would be like Simeon, the man that you allowed to live until he saw the Messiah, Jesus Christ. You are not slack concerning your promises. My life is not cursed as I might think it is. You love me enough to wean me off this world."

Chapter 5
AND TURN FROM THEIR WICKED WAYS

A few months before her death, Allie is sitting with Dr. Schultz in a hospital exam room. Allie is sitting on the bed, and Dr. Schultz is sitting in a chair.

Dr. Schultz said, "Ms. Black, I don't have a cure for the sickness inside you. I don't know how to take away your discomfort or heal you. Nonetheless, I can prescribe some medication to you that can try to slow down the virus' aggression and prolong your life. Would you like to try this medication?"

Allie replied, "Dr. Schultz, I thank you for everything that you do and try to do for my health. However, I will consult a physician of higher authority."

Dr. Schultz asked, "Okay. Good. Would you like me to call him or her and give my personal recommendation? Who is this, other doctor?

Allie replied, "Do you believe this doctor can cure the virus and heal me? If you don't believe, there is no need to ask him. His name is Jesus Christ."

Dr. Schultz said, "I see. I was raised in the church also. I know Jesus."

Allie replied, "That's good. But, even better, does He know you?"

Dr. Schultz said, "I would hope so. I spent most of my life trying to help other people. This is why I become a doctor."

Allie said, "Sir, our righteousness is as filthy rags. The only way that Jesus knows you is by His Spirit. You must be born again."

Dr. Schultz replied, "I heard about that from the preacher during the altar calls. I went up to the altar and gave my life to Christ and told him how sorry I was for my sins."

Allie said, "It is not enough to be sorry for your sins. You must repent, be baptized by the water in the name of Jesus Christ for the remission of sins and receive the Holy Ghost with the evidence to speak in other tongues as the Spirit of God gives the utterance."

Dr. Schultz replied, "I heard teachings on speaking in tongues. But, isn't tongues just a gift that only some people have?"

Allie said, "When a baby is born of his mother, he cries or speaks in a language for his mother. When you are born of God, you cry for your Father or speak in other tongues for your Father. Nobody else teaches the baby to cry for his mother in another language. And, nobody else shall teach you to cry for God in another language."

Dr. Schultz replied, "I guess I'm not born again. I will start working on this soon. And, you start working on getting better."

Allie said, "Yes, doctor. Jesus has been working on my healing ever since I ask him to heal me. You see, sir. In order for us to be healed of an aggressive sickness and disease as this one, we must agree to put our lives in Jesus' hands. And, we must put our lives in his hands. Jesus will let the virus run its course in my body in order to exhaust its strength, so it can't fight anymore. Then, Jesus will purge the virus from me. I must be put to sleep and opened, so God's army, the locusts and worms, can consume the bacterium on my body, organs, tissues and cells and consume also the viruses in the cells. This will take some time, but I am willing to wait. Besides, I am sleeping. I can do nothing else but wait on the Lord."

Dr. Schultz replied, "But, Ms. Black. Doesn't God help us when we help ourselves?"

Allie said, "I am helping myself by going to a physician with more knowledge, skills and experience to do the job. I went to you and other physicians on Earth, and you told me that you could not cure the condition or heal me. Now, if I did not want to help myself, I would refuse to call on the Lord for help. I would be content to just live with the virus and fight a losing battle with inferior medication. This brings me to my next point. Another requirement for healing is to turn from our wicked ways. Isaiah, a prophet of God, wrote that God's ways are not our ways. His thoughts are not our thoughts. Human beings can see only so far into the past and future, but God can see all the way to the beginning and ending. He is Alpha and Omega, the beginning and ending and the first and last. Are you ready to believe, Mr. Schultz?"

Dr. Schultz replied, "I admire your faith, Allie, despite your circumstances. But, I'm still trying to wrap my head around how this condition can be cured. I know God has all power, but how does He heal?"

Allie said, "Doc, you must seek God's face. God is a Spirit.

God cannot be found in natural things. God is not in medication and scientific machines. We must come out of ourselves in order to see God's face. When we see God's face, we will see His way."

Dr. Schultz replied, "Allie, I was in school for many years and excelled in every class, but the understanding that came through your lips was far superior than the academic knowledge I received from school."

Allie said, "School is good. Education is good, but man's wisdom is not the final frontier. God put two major trees in the garden of Eden. Those were the tree of life and tree of the knowledge of good and evil. The tree of life is Jesus Christ. Jesus is the serpent that eats the other serpents. Jesus is the King Snake. Viruses are little serpents inside cells. Jesus is the Resurrection also. Life is in Jesus. Jesus has the ability to consume the infected cells and blood and create new cells and blood to give a person more life. We try to use the inferior snakes to heal us. To illustrate, we use parts of viruses and make vaccines in order to protect us from other viruses. I appreciate your services in the healthcare profession, Dr. Schultz, but I desire to stay with Jesus."

Chapter 6
THEN WILL I HEAR FROM HEAVEN

Ali is driving his car on Interstate 55 to Memphis from New Orleans. Ali was on the road by daybreak. He's driving a red 2000 Saturn. Ali is not moving; he's just driving in order to change the scenery a little. Ali has New Orleans in his blood; he can't move. In addition, New Orleans has Allie's body. In saying this, Ali wants to be there when the Lord Jesus Christ awakens her from surgery in perfect health. Ali has been prophesying about the special miracle to many, other people. Some of them believe him, but others don't. Nonetheless, they respect his beliefs and don't try to discourage him. On another note, the traffic is moderate, and the clouds are thick and gray. The temperature is cool with some wind. It begins to rain, and the rain increases. Furthermore, it rains for an hour. Nevertheless, Ali continues to drive through the rain and listen to gospel music on a radio station. Ali keeps his eyes on the road. He makes sure that he reads all the signs to Memphis. Diligence and attention to detail make a good watchman.

If Ali does not watch and pray, he will fail to see this special miracle and the rapture. Ali sings with the music on the radio. Ali sings to God, however. Ali remembers that Allie loves to sing. In addition, he loves to hear her sing. The rain passes from East to West and leaves the area. Plus, the clouds begin to open, and the sunlight is revealed from the heavens. Ali smiles at the glorious sight because it is a sign that God hears the call from Allie and him about her health. Ali imagines to hear angels sing, "Hallelujah, holy, holy, holy, Lord God Almighty who was, and is, and is to come. Holy, Holy, Holy to the Highest." Angelic voices give confirmation. Human voices just give sensation. Therefore, human voices appeal to the five senses and can make the body move, but angelic voices comfort the soul of a person. The soul is the mediator with the mind and spirit. The soul transports and translates messages from the spirit to the mind. Angels deposit words into a person's spirit which translation comforts the soul and is understood by the mind.

Therefore, faith is an inner confidence
even though the body might show concern
at the circumstances in his life. As
Ali drives to Memphis, he thinks about
the good and bad times that Allie and
he endure together. To illustrate, Ali
recalls the stimulating conversations
at the restaurants, the quiet times at
the movies, the intimacies during
kisses and the distress from the
sickness and the circumstances of the
sickness. Some of the memories cause
Ali to shed tears like Jesus sheds His
blood for the remission of our sins.
The Roman soldiers bruised Jesus' body
by a whip, and blood was shed. On the
other hand, the loss of Allie bruised
Ali's soul to cause him to shed tears.
In addition, the Roman soldiers put a
crown of thorns on Jesus' head, and the
thorns pierced His skin to shed blood.
Hence, the memory of Allie's life,
sickness and death brings Ali to shed
tears. Furthermore, the Roman soldiers
pierced Jesus with a sword in His side,
so that the Lord shed blood and water.
Therefore, the angry words from other
people at the sight of Allie's
condition against Ali cause emotional
discomfort. In addition, Ali sheds
tears.

Ali is experiencing the crucifixion of Jesus Christ in another form. After Jesus suffered a while, He was ready to give up the ghost. Nonetheless, Jesus did not die until He helped the helpless. Thus, Ali has become more helpful after Allie's death. Allie's legacy has made Ali a better man. Allie would be proud of Ali's maturity even through grief. God is restoring Ali as He is restoring Allie. Ali and Allie are so close spiritually that God allows Ali to feel His healing power in Allie. Ali feels the purging of Allie's body. Ali feels the tingling of the balm of the anointing oil of the Holy Ghost in Allie's body. Furthermore, Ali will feel her resurrection. This is love. This is the intimacy between a man and woman. On the other hand, Ali is going through Jackson, and he decides to stop at a restaurant to refuel his body. In the restaurant, Ali is sitting at a table for two beside another man that is considerably older than Ali is. This man's name is Jack.

Jack said, "Howdy, partner. How you doing?"

Ali replied, "I'm making it, sir. How about yourself?"

Jack said, "I'm wonderful. We had some good rain earlier, but it looks like it done cleared up a bit, eh."

Ali replied, "Sure has. I drove through much of it."

Jack said, "Is that right? By the way, my name is Jack."

Ali replied, "Ali. Nice to meet you."

Jack said, "Same here. So, where you headed?"

Ali replied, "Memphis."

Jack said, "That's a big city. You have family there? Friends?"

Ali replied, "Nah. Just traveling. It's no bigger than New Orleans."

Jack said, "So, you're from the N.O., eh. I worked on a towboat in New Orleans for many years."

Ali replied, "Yeah. They have a lot of those down there. How is it like to work on a towboat?"

Jack said, "It's basically a floating house. You get a chance to become a family with the crew."

Ali replied, "Oh. I see."

Jack said, "Speaking of family. Are you in the family of God?"

Ali replied, "Yes. I am born again, born of the water and Spirit."

Jack said, "That's good because Jesus Christ is coming back really soon. He is going to return in the same manner that He comes the first time. I mean Jesus is going to come back to fulfill all the calls for healing from His people even from some of the dead ones before He takes His people up."

Chapter 7
AND FORGIVE THEIR SINS

Six feet deep in the earth is a body in a cushioned casket. Her clothes are dry rotted from her body. Her body stinks. The LORD sends his army of cankerworms and taper worms to Allie's body for decomposition. The worms work like a highly skilled surgical team. The worms open Allie's flesh and break down her infected body. Allie's condition shall remain anonymous, but the viruses in her blood infected the rest of her body. Therefore, in order to restore Allie's health, the cells; tissues and organs must be replaced with new ones. It's like how an auto mechanic breaks down an engine to replace the parts and restore the motor to full capability. These worms work tirelessly; however. They don't get paid. They are made to obey the commandments of the living God, and they obey better than humans obey. Tearing down a human body and rebuilding it is a tedious task. Thus, the worms have to be dedicated to the mission in order to accomplish it.

In this God-made surgical room, there
is no room for mistakes because God is
perfect. In addition, human error and
ignorance are not factors because God
is in complete control. Above the
grave, similar missions are being
accomplished by humans on smaller
scales. For example, demolition crews
are tearing down a 100-year old home in
order to build a new one in its place.
Everybody is safety conscious from the
superintendant to the general laborer.
Yet, the demolition crews cannot work
outside the house in the rain.
However, the worms work in the rain,
sleet, snow, hail, heat, freeze and so
on. On the other hand, the owners of
this house, the Miller's, are waiting
in a temporary lodging until their
house is restored. Hence, Allie is
waiting in paradise until the LORD
Jesus Christ and His worms restore and
resurrect her body into perfect health.
What does it cost people to hire God to
restore their bodies to perfect health?
Faith in God is the price for miracles
and special miracles. Nonetheless, it
will cost the Miller's $1,000,000 to
tear down the old home and rebuild it
with new materials. God says that He
builds us from the dust of the ground.
In saying this, Allie's body is in the
right place for healing. Somewhere
above ground, Ali is going about his
life and waiting on the LORD.

33

The Earth's surface is a waiting room for the loved ones that want desperately to see the restoration and resurrection of their dear friends. To the contrary, only faith in God will please Him to do this task. Meanwhile, six feet deep in the earth in a cushioned casket, the worms continue to be diligent and hymn a song from their moist skins.

The worms sing, "Rebuilding the temple for our LORD. Rebuilding the temple is not hard. Rebuilding the temple with pride and grace. Rebuilding the temple is not a race. Rebuilding the temple to put a smile on somebody's face. Rebuilding the temple is our case. Rebuilding the temple for the glory of God. Rebuilding the temple under a merciful rod. Rebuilding the temples of the rich and the poor. Rebuilding the temple from the roof to the floor. Rebuilding the temple with no money or credit. Rebuilding the temple, and then, He'll sell it. He will sell it for faith and submission to His will. Rebuilding the temple beneath a hill. Rebuilding the temple for the love of God's people.

Rebuilding the temple without a
steeple. Rebuilding the temple
according to God's instructions.
Rebuilding the temple, so this woman
can function. Rebuilding the temple
for a testimony of healing.
Rebuilding the temple with a hard
ceiling. Rebuilding the temple without
Satan to interfere. Rebuilding the
temple without fear."

On another note, in the library,
Ali begins to sing to himself as he
lies on a sofa, cradles a book with his
hands to his breastplate and looks to
the ceiling.

Ali sings, "O LORD, you are so
mighty. O LORD, you are so great. O
LORD, you are so mighty. O LORD, you
shall heal my mate. O LORD, you are so
mighty. O LORD, you are so great. O
LORD, you are so mighty. O LORD,
health is our fate. O LORD, you are so
mighty. O LORD, you are so great. O
LORD, you are so mighty. You are the
love that conquers hate. O LORD, you
are so mighty. O LORD, you are so
great. O LORD, you are so mighty. O
LORD, you are healing her with fish
bait. O LORD, you are so mighty. O
LORD, you are so great. O LORD, you
are so mighty. O LORD, your miracles
are worth the wait. O LORD, you are so
mighty. O LORD, you are so great. O
LORD, you are so mighty.

You're right on time; you're never late."

Ali rises from his seat and stands on his feet. Ali puts the book back in its place on the shelf. Ali walks out of the library with a smile of faith, but the sorrow of the loss of Allie is buried deep in his mind. Nonetheless, Ali continues to study Journalism at Tulane. Later, Ali is walking in the park and sees Jack. They meet and shake each other's hands.

Jack said, "Hi, buddy. How you doing?"

Ali replied, "I'm okay. How are you? What's up?"

Jack said, "I was just going over some verses in Joel with the LORD about how He pities His people and promises to restore the years that the locusts, cankerworms and taper worms have eaten."

Ali replied, "Yes, sir. I was just singing to the LORD about the same thing. We see God at work in the secret place. But, the world can't see His works. Neither will they see the finished product. They are blind with two, healthy eyes."

Jack said, "Yep. And, they don't even realize that before the LORD takes us up into Heaven, He will perform many miracles and special miracles to fulfill the many demands of faith from His people."

36

Chapter 8
AND HEAL THE LAND

Ali lies in his bed and envisions the time that he is a boy and looks down at the ants on its mound. Then, Ali remembers the verses in Proverbs 6 about the ants. Hence, Ali thinks about an innumerable number of ants bringing new flesh to Allie's body and stacking it to get ready to put the new flesh together with the old and new flesh. The ants are working like a construction crew. The Holy Bible states that the ants are not strong, but they are diligent. Lying on his bed and watching each ant put little pieces of flesh back into Allie's body makes Ali go to sleep. Nonetheless, the ants still work while Ali sleeps. Ali is sitting on a park bench the next morning and watching the construction crews slowly but steadily replace the old materials with new materials on an existing building.

Ali said, "I never saw an ant sweat, but we sweat. I never saw an ant take a water break, but we take water breaks. I never saw an ant late for work, but we are late for work. I never saw an ant leave work early, but we leave work early.

I never saw an ant get fired, but we
get fired. I never saw an ant stay
home from work, but we stay home from
work. The ants are way better workers
than we are. God wants us to take
advice from them. We should give the
ants advice. However, the ants give us
advice. We have overseers, but the
ants don't need overseers. The ants
are self-motivated to get the job done.
That's what I call hard. The ants are
hard, but we just talk hard in rap
videos. We show off our big muscles
and tattoos and think that makes us
hard. The ants have neither of these
things, but they are born to be hard."

Ali continues to watch the
construction workers. In saying this,
they built a scaffold to the top of the
building that is not very high. Each
level of the scaffold has two men.
They are laying the bricks to the outer
structure of the building. On humans,
the skin is the bricks. God put new
skins on Adam and Eve to cover their
nakedness. Jesus' body is eternal.
Jesus regenerates Himself. Jesus is
the Lamb of God. God takes skin off of
Jesus' body and stretches it out like a
baker rolls out the dough.

God gives the elastic skin to the ants
to carry it to Allie's body and put it
on her. God is a Spirit. God moves
like the wind moves. Ali looks at
another college student sitting on the
bench, and the pages of her book are
turning by the wind. The skin of our
body is like a scroll. God's Spirit
rolls out a part of Jesus' skin, and
Jesus' skin has the word of God in it.
This is why Jesus is called the Word of
God. Therefore, the Word of God
becomes a part of Allie. Furthermore,
what word of God will other people read
in Allie? How about this one: I am
the resurrection and the life. He that
believes in me, once he was dead, yet
shall he live. In addition, Allie's
body shall read, "If my people which
are called by my name shall humble
themselves and pray, and seek my face,
and turn from their wicked ways, then
will I hear from heaven, and forgive
their sins, and heal their land."
Nevertheless, the young woman that sits
on the bench with Ali is Martha.

Ali said, "Hello, my name is Ali.
How are you?"

Martha replied, "Hey, I'm Martha.
Fine."

Ali asked, "What are you reading?"

Martha replied, "I'm studying for
a science test."

Ali asked, "Wow. Is science your
favorite subject?"

Martha replied, "Sure is."

Ali asked, "What's your major?

Martha replied, "Bioengineering."

Ali asked, "So, you want to know how the human body is built, eh?"

Martha replied, "Somewhat. But, my main focus is on the restoration of the body after it is purged of viruses, such as HIV and Ebola."

Ali asked, "What have you learned so far?"

Martha replied, "I learned that all the fundraisers in the world could not find a cure for HIV and Ebola. The cure comes only from Jesus Christ."

Ali said, "Amen, sister."

Martha replied, "I take it you're a Christian."

Ali said, "Yes, madme. I am born again."

Martha replied, "You don't have to call me madme, sir. Even though, I appreciate the respect."

Ali asked, "You're welcomed, Martha. Do you want to take a study break and get some lunch?"

Martha replied, "Is this a date, Ali?"

Ali said, "Nah, just lunch. I can use the company."

Thus, Ali and Martha get up from the park bench and walk out of the park across the crosswalk and into an Italian restaurant across the street. Martha made sure that all her books were in the book bag. Ali opens the door for Martha, and she walks into the restaurant first.

Martha said, "Thank you."

Ali walked into the restaurant behind Martha and let the door close softly.

Ali replied, "You're welcomed."

A waitress meets Ali and Martha at the receptionist's desk.

Waitress asked, "Good afternoon, welcome to Cambroni's. Where do you want to sit, in the center or by the window?"

Ali replied, "By the window, please."

Ali and Martha follow the waitress to a table by the window in the back of the restaurant because the other tables by the window are being used. The waitress holds out her right hand to the seats, and Ali lets Martha go to her seat by the window first. Ali holds the chair out a little for Martha.

Martha said, "Thank you."

Then, Ali sits in his seat.

Waitress asked, "Would you like something to drink?"

41

Martha replied, "Water, please. Thank you."

Ali replied, "Sprite, please. Thank you."

Waitress said, "You're welcomed. Take your time and look at the menu, and I'll be back to take your dinner order."

Ali and Martha nodded their heads and smiled, and the waitress walked away gracefully with a smile.

www.ingramcontent.com/pod-product-compliance
Lightning Source LLC
Chambersburg PA
CBHW070507290526
45790CB00003B/1128